Juicing for Kidney Rejuvenation

Ultimate guide and recipes to a balanced and healthy lifestyle.

Rupert L Crane

Copyright © 2024 by Rupert L. Crane

Table of content

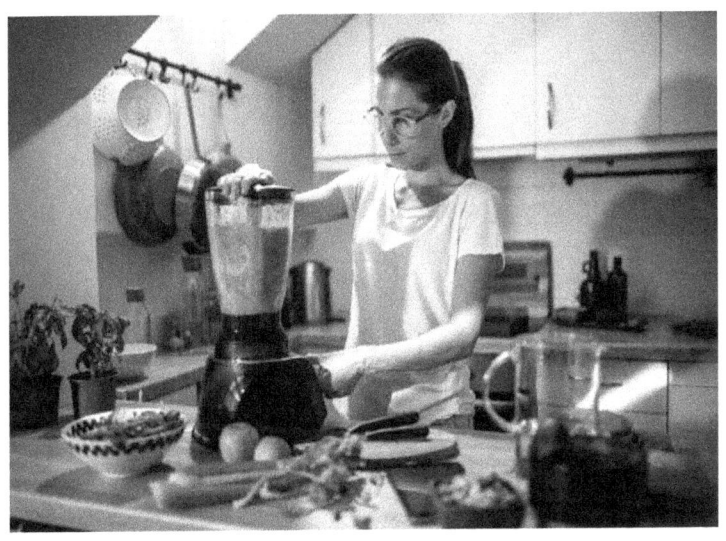

Introduction

Unveiling the transformative potential of juicing for kidney health.

Our bodies, intricate and harmonious, are a symphony of systems working in tandem to maintain equilibrium and sustain life. Among these unsung heroes, the kidneys stand out as silent sentinels, performing a role so vital that their significance often goes unnoticed until they falter. The importance of kidney health cannot be overstated, as these bean-shaped organs play a pivotal role in maintaining the delicate balance necessary for the body's optimal functioning.

At their core, the kidneys are natural filtration units, purifying the bloodstream by removing waste, excess fluids, and electrolytes. They act as the body's detoxifiers, ensuring that harmful substances are expelled while essential elements are retained. Beyond this, the kidneys contribute to the regulation of blood pressure, the production of red blood cells, and the activation of vitamin D, underlining their multi-faceted importance.

When our kidneys operate smoothly, their silent efficiency often goes unnoticed. However, when kidney function is compromised, a cascade of health issues can unfold. Chronic kidney disease, kidney stones, infections, and other renal disorders can emerge, impacting not only the kidneys themselves but also exerting systemic effects on the entire body. Elevated blood pressure, anemia, and compromised bone health are just a few repercussions of impaired kidney function, highlighting the interconnected nature of our physiological systems.

The rise in kidney-related ailments in recent years signals a need for a proactive and holistic approach to kidney health. Lifestyle factors, environmental stressors, and dietary choices contribute to the burden placed on our kidneys, emphasizing the urgency of adopting practices that support and rejuvenate these vital filters.

Juicing as a Natural Approach to Support Kidney Function: A Fresh Perspective

In the quest for optimal health, the concept of using juicing as a natural approach to support kidney function emerges as a beacon of hope and possibility. Juicing, the art of extracting the pure essence from fruits, vegetables, and herbs, offers a refreshing departure from conventional approaches to kidney health. It represents a harmonious alliance between nature's bounty and the intricate needs of our renal system.

At its core, juicing embodies simplicity and purity. It is a celebration of the vibrant hues of nature's produce, a liquid manifestation of the nutrients that fortify and heal. The transformative potential of juicing lies not just in its taste and refreshment but in the concentrated dose of vitamins, minerals, and antioxidants it delivers.

As we delve into the realm of juicing for kidney health, it is crucial to recognize that this is not a mere culinary trend but a profound shift toward embracing the therapeutic power of whole foods. The fruits and vegetables selected for juicing are not arbitrary; they are chosen with precision, aligning with the nutritional needs of our kidneys. The goal is not just to create palatable beverages but to craft elixirs that specifically target kidney support and rejuvenation.

One of the primary advantages of juicing lies in its potential to alleviate the burden on the kidneys. Unlike solid foods, which require digestion and processing, juices offer a readily absorbed form of nutrition. This liquid form allows the body to extract essential nutrients efficiently, reducing the workload on the kidneys and facilitating their natural detoxification processes.

Moreover, juicing provides a concentrated source of hydration, a critical aspect of kidney health. Staying adequately hydrated is essential for the kidneys to flush out waste products and maintain the optimal balance of electrolytes. Juices, infused with the hydrating essence of fruits and vegetables, become a delicious and effective means of supporting the kidneys in their regulatory functions.

The concept of using juicing for kidney health is not an isolated practice; it integrates seamlessly into a holistic approach to well-being. It is not a replacement for medical interventions when necessary but rather a complementary strategy that empowers individuals to take an active role in their health. Juicing becomes a catalyst for lifestyle changes, encouraging the adoption of nutritious diets, regular exercise, and stress management practices—cornerstones of kidney health.

In the chapters that follow, we will unravel the nuances of juicing for kidney rejuvenation. We will explore the specific nutrients that contribute to kidney health, master the art of crafting purposeful and delicious juices, and delve into the broader aspects of a lifestyle that fosters resilience. The Power of Juicing for Kidney Rejuvenation is not just a guide; it is an invitation to embark on a transformative journey—one where the simplicity of juicing converges with the profound needs of our kidneys, unlocking a path to sustained well-being and vitality.

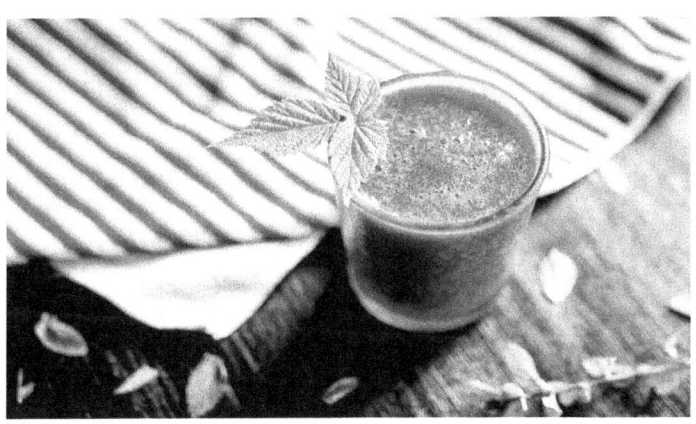

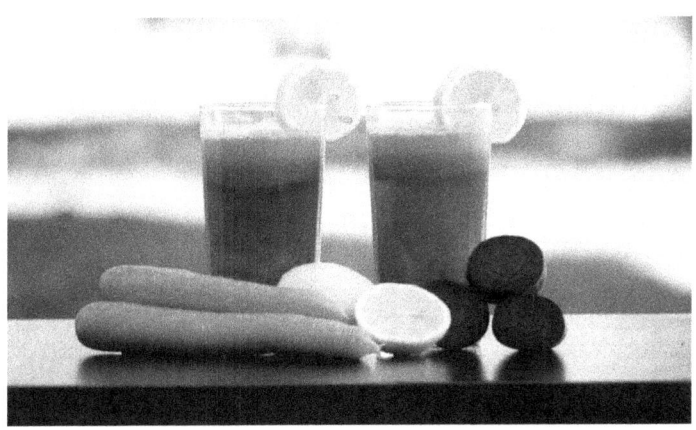

CHAPTER 1

Understanding Kidney Health

Understanding Kidney Health: Nurturing the Vital Filters

The human body, a marvel of intricate design, relies on a symphony of organs and systems to maintain equilibrium and sustain life. Among these, the kidneys emerge as unsung heroes, performing a crucial role that extends far beyond what meets the eye. To comprehend the essence of kidney health, one must embark on a journey into the intricate workings of these bean-shaped organs and explore the common issues and diseases that can disrupt their delicate balance.

The Renal Symphony: The Role of Kidneys in the Body

Nestled in the small of the back, just beneath the ribcage, the kidneys function as the body's natural filtration system. Picture them as meticulous custodians, tirelessly working to purify the bloodstream and maintain a delicate equilibrium within the body.

The primary responsibility of the kidneys is to filter waste products and excess fluids from the blood, creating urine as a byproduct. This process, occurring continuously, ensures that harmful substances are expelled from the body, preventing the accumulation of toxins. Simultaneously, the kidneys play a pivotal role in maintaining the balance of essential elements, such as sodium, potassium, and calcium, critical for overall health.

Beyond their role as filters, the kidneys are integral to various physiological processes. They produce erythropoietin, a hormone that stimulates the production of red blood cells in the bone marrow. This function contributes to the body's ability to transport oxygen effectively. Additionally, the kidneys are key players in regulating blood pressure. Through the intricate interplay of hormones and fluid balance, they help control the volume of blood circulating through the body, influencing blood pressure levels.

Moreover, the kidneys are essential for activating vitamin D, a crucial element for the absorption of calcium in the intestines. This function not only supports bone health but also has far-reaching effects on the immune system and overall well-being.

In essence, the kidneys serve as vigilant guardians, maintaining a delicate balance that is fundamental to the body's optimal functioning. Their significance extends beyond filtration, encompassing the regulation of blood pressure, production of red blood cells, and facilitation of vitamin D activation.

Common Kidney-Related Issues and Diseases

Despite their resilience and efficiency, kidneys are not immune to challenges. The modern lifestyle, laden with processed foods, environmental pollutants, and high stress levels, has contributed to the rise of kidney-related issues. Understanding these common challenges is essential for fostering kidney health and well-being.

Chronic Kidney Disease (CKD):

CKD is a condition which occurs when the kidney losses function gradually over time. It often develops silently, with symptoms manifesting in later stages. Diabetes, hypertension, and aging are common contributing factors to CKD.

Kidney Stones:

These are hard deposits that form in the kidneys when urine contains high levels of certain substances, such as calcium, oxalate, and phosphorus. The formation of kidney stones can cause excruciating pain and may result in complications if not addressed promptly.

Urinary Tract Infections (UTIs):

UTI t affect any part of the urinary, which also includes the kidneys. UTIs can lead to inflammation, discomfort, and, if left untreated, may progress to more severe kidney infections.

Polycystic Kidney Disease (PKD):

A genetic disorder characterized by the formation of fluid-filled cysts in the kidneys. These cysts can interfere with kidney function and, over time, lead to kidney failure.

Acute Kidney Injury (AKI):

A sudden and often reversible loss of kidney function typically caused by factors such as dehydration, severe infection, or medication side effects. AKI requires prompt medical attention.

Hypertension (High Blood Pressure):

Prolonged high blood pressure can damage the blood vessels in the kidneys, reducing their ability to function properly. Conversely, impaired kidney function can contribute to elevated blood pressure, creating a cyclical relationship.

Glomerulonephritis:

Inflammation of the glomeruli, the tiny blood vessels in the kidneys responsible for filtration. This condition can be acute or chronic, affecting kidney function and potentially leading to kidney failure. Intervention and the formulation of effective preventive strategies. Regular health check-ups, maintaining a healthy lifestyle, and addressing risk factors promptly contribute to the overall well-being of the kidneys.

CHAPTER 2

Nutrition for Kidney Health

In the intricate dance of well-being, nutrition takes center stage, especially when it comes to the health of our vital filters—the kidneys. Crafting a kidney-friendly diet is not merely a culinary endeavor but a deliberate and conscious choice to support these resilient organs. Let's embark on a journey through the elements of a kidney-friendly diet, exploring the nutrients that fortify and the dietary strategies that nurture.

Kidney-Friendly Diet: Balancing Nutrients for Resilience

Manage Protein Intake:

While protein is a crucial component for overall health, excessive protein consumption can strain the kidneys. In a kidney-friendly diet, it's essential to strike a balance. High-quality protein sources like fish, poultry, eggs, and plant-based proteins can be incorporated in moderate amounts, ensuring adequate nutrition without overburdening the kidneys.

Control Phosphorus and Potassium:

Kidneys play a pivotal role in regulating phosphorus and potassium levels in the body. In kidney-related conditions, such as chronic kidney disease (CKD), these minerals can become imbalanced. Foods rich in phosphorus, such as dairy products, nuts, and seeds, should be consumed in moderation. Similarly, managing potassium intake by limiting high-potassium foods like bananas, oranges, and potatoes is crucial.

Monitor Sodium Intake:

Sodium, which is frequently present in processed meals and table salt, can lead to fluid retention and high blood pressure. A kidney-friendly diet emphasizes the moderation of sodium intake. Choosing fresh, whole foods and using herbs and spices for flavoring instead of excessive salt can help manage sodium levels effectively.

Emphasize Heart-Healthy Fats:

Opting for heart-healthy fats, such as those found in avocados, olive oil, and fatty fish, supports overall cardiovascular health. This is particularly important as cardiovascular health is intricately linked to kidney health.

Include Adequate Fiber:

A diet rich in fiber promotes digestive health and helps regulate blood sugar levels. Whole grains, fruits, vegetables, and legumes contribute to a kidney-friendly diet while providing essential nutrients and fiber.

Moderate Fluid Intake:

While hydration is essential, individuals with compromised kidney function may need to monitor their fluid intake. The specific recommendations may vary based on individual health conditions. Consulting with a healthcare professional is crucial to determine appropriate fluid levels.

Limit Sugar and Refined Carbohydrates:

Excessive sugar and refined carbohydrates can contribute to weight gain and blood sugar fluctuations, potentially impacting kidney health. A kidney-friendly diet encourages the moderation of sugar intake and the preference for complex carbohydrates.

It's important to note that the ideal kidney-friendly diet may vary based on individual health conditions and the stage of kidney disease. Therefore, consulting with a healthcare provider or a registered dietitian is essential to tailor dietary recommendations to specific needs.

In essence, a kidney-friendly diet revolves around balance and moderation. It aims to provide essential nutrients while managing the intake of substances that might burden the kidneys. This dietary approach supports overall health, reduces the risk of complications, and contributes to the resilience of these vital organs.

Nourishing with Fluids : Importances

Beyond the composition of nutrients, the role of hydration stands as a cornerstone in the realm of kidney health. Adequate fluid intake is not just a matter of quenching thirst; it is a vital component of maintaining the delicate balance within the kidneys.

Optimal Filtration and Waste Removal:

Hydration facilitates the filtration process within the kidneys. A well-hydrated body ensures that waste products are effectively flushed out through urine, preventing the build-up of toxins that can compromise kidney function.

Prevention of Kidney Stones:

Ample fluid intake reduces the concentration of minerals in the urine, lowering the risk of kidney stone formation. Dehydration can lead to the crystallization of minerals, potentially causing painful kidney stones.

Blood Pressure Regulation:

Proper hydration supports blood volume and helps regulate blood pressure. Maintaining stable blood pressure is crucial for the health of blood vessels in the kidneys.

Temperature Regulation and Electrolyte Balance:

Hydration plays a role in regulating body temperature and ensuring the balance of electrolytes, including sodium and potassium. These factors are integral to overall kidney health.

Prevention of Urinary Tract Infections (UTIs):

Hydration supports the flushing of bacteria from the urinary tract, reducing the risk of urinary tract infections that can affect the kidneys.

While hydration is undeniably important, individual needs may vary. Factors such as age, climate, physical activity, and health conditions can influence the optimal amount of fluid intake. As a general guideline, aiming for around eight 8-ounce glasses of water per day is a common recommendation, but adjusting based on individual requirements is key.

CHAPTER 3

The Benefits of Juicing For Kidneys

Juicing offers a nutrient-dense and hydrating elixir that supports kidney health through antioxidant protection, anti-inflammatory effects, and the promotion of optimal hydration. By harnessing the nutritional benefits of different fruits and vegetables, individuals can embark on a journey to nourish and fortify their vital filters, fostering resilience and well-being.

Let's delve into the manifold benefits of juicing for kidneys, exploring the nutritional treasures that various fruits and vegetables bring to the table.

1. Hydration Support:
Adequate hydration is crucial for kidney health, as it facilitates the flushing out of toxins and waste products. Juicing provides a delicious and hydrating way to meet fluid needs, infusing the body with the water content present in fruits and vegetables. Cucumber, watermelon, and citrus

fruits are excellent choices for their high water content, contributing to optimal hydration.

2. Antioxidant Boost:

Antioxidants play a pivotal role in combating oxidative stress, a factor that can contribute to kidney damage. Fruits and vegetables, particularly berries, leafy greens, and citrus fruits, are rich in antioxidants such as vitamin C, flavonoids, and polyphenols. These compounds help neutralize free radicals, supporting the overall health of the kidneys.

3. Anti-Inflammatory Properties:

Chronic inflammation is a common contributor to kidney diseases. Juicing with ingredients like ginger and turmeric, known for their anti-inflammatory properties, provides a natural and flavorful way to help manage inflammation, potentially protecting the kidneys from harm.

4. Nutrient Density:

Juicing allows for the extraction of concentrated nutrients from a variety of fruits and vegetables. Leafy greens like kale and spinach are powerhouses of vitamins A and K, essential for maintaining healthy kidney function. The inclusion of a diverse range of produce ensures a spectrum of nutrients that contribute to overall well-being.

5. Blood Pressure Regulation:

One of the main risk factors for renal disorders is high blood pressure.. Beets, known for their nitrate content, have been linked to lower blood pressure. Juicing with beets and other nitrate-rich vegetables may contribute to blood pressure regulation, providing a protective effect for the kidneys.

6. Kidney Detoxification:

Certain fruits and vegetables, such as lemons and cranberries, have natural diuretic properties. Incorporating these into juices can support the kidneys in flushing out toxins and promoting detoxification, fostering a healthier internal environment.

7. pH Balance:

Maintaining a slightly alkaline pH in the body is believed to be beneficial for kidney health. Juicing with alkaline-forming fruits and vegetables, including leafy greens, cucumber, and celery, may contribute to a more alkaline state, supporting the kidneys in their regulatory functions.

8. Potassium Regulation:

Individuals with kidney issues often need to manage their potassium intake. Juicing allows for careful selection of fruits and vegetables with moderate potassium content, such as apples, berries, and carrots, contributing to a kidney-friendly balance.

9. Improved Nutrient Absorption:

The liquid form of juices allows for easier absorption of nutrients, offering a more efficient way for the body to assimilate essential vitamins and minerals. This can be particularly beneficial for individuals with compromised kidney function who may struggle with nutrient absorption from solid foods.

10. Flavorful Variety and Adherence to Dietary Restrictions:

Juicing provides a creative and enjoyable way to incorporate a variety of fruits and vegetables into the diet. For individuals with dietary restrictions or aversions, juicing can be a palatable and convenient solution, ensuring a diverse intake of nutrients.

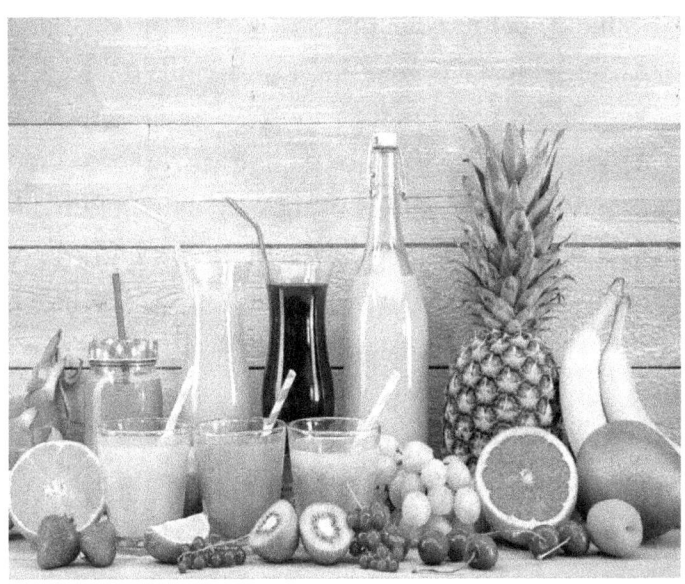

CHAPTER 4

Selecting the Right ingredients

When embarking on the journey of juicing for kidney health, selecting the right ingredients is paramount. Choosing kidney-friendly fruits and vegetables ensures that your elixirs are not only delicious but also nourishing for these vital organs. Let's explore a curated list of kidney-friendly ingredients, delving into the nutritional content of each to craft a symphony of wellness.

1. Cucumber:

Nutritional Content: Cucumbers are hydrating and low in potassium, making them an excellent base for kidney-friendly juices. They contain vitamins K and C, as well as antioxidants like beta-carotene. Cucumbers contribute to hydration and provide a refreshing flavor to your juices.

2. Watermelon:

Nutritional Content: With its high water content, watermelon is a hydrating and kidney-friendly fruit. It contains vitamins A and C, along with antioxidants like lycopene. Watermelon adds natural sweetness to juices without burdening the kidneys with excessive potassium.

3. Berries (Blueberries, Strawberries, Raspberries):

Nutritional Content: Berries are rich in antioxidants, particularly vitamin C and flavonoids. They offer a burst of flavor without contributing significant potassium, making them an excellent choice for kidney-friendly juicing. Berries also provide fiber, promoting digestive health.

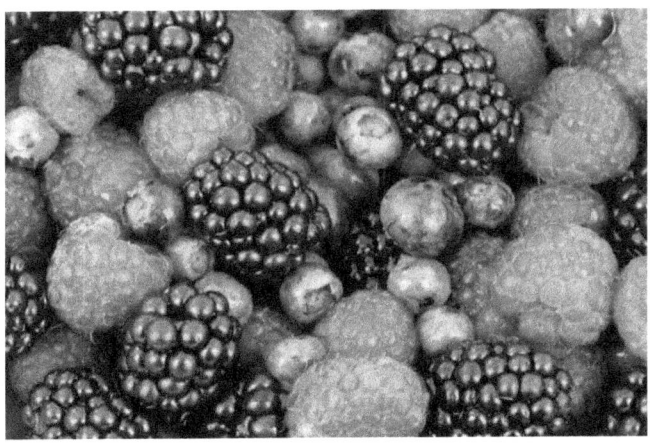

4. Apples:

Nutritional Content: Apples are low in potassium and high in fiber, making them kidney-friendly. They contain vitamin C and various antioxidants. Apples add sweetness and a pleasant crunch to your juices without compromising renal health.

5. Pineapple:

Nutritional Content: Pineapple is a tropical delight that adds sweetness to juices. Contains an enzyme with anti-inflammatory properties called bromelain. While moderately high in potassium, pineapple can be enjoyed in moderation, providing a unique flavor profile.

6. Red Grapes:

Nutritional Content: Red grapes, in addition to being delicious, contain resveratrol, an antioxidant with potential anti-inflammatory effects. They are lower in potassium compared to other fruits like bananas, making them suitable for kidney-friendly juicing.

7. Kale:

Nutritional Content: Kale is a nutrient powerhouse, offering vitamins A, C, and K, along with minerals like iron and calcium. It is low in potassium and adds a hearty, earthy flavor to your juices. Kale contributes to overall health while being kind to the kidneys.

8. Spinach:

Nutritional Content: Spinach is a versatile leafy green rich in vitamins A and K. It is low in potassium, making it a kidney-friendly ingredient. Spinach adds a mild, slightly sweet taste to juices while providing essential nutrients.

9. Carrots:

Nutritional Content: Carrots are a good source of beta-carotene, a precursor to vitamin A. They are low in potassium and add natural sweetness to juices. Carrots contribute to eye health and provide a vibrant orange hue to your concoctions.

10. Celery:

Nutritional Content: Celery is a hydrating and low-potassium vegetable. It adds a crisp, refreshing flavor to juices. Celery is also rich in antioxidants and may have anti-inflammatory properties, supporting overall well-being.

Extras for your dedication to your rejuvenation journey;

11. Cranberries:

Nutritional Content: Cranberries are known for their tart flavor and potential benefits for urinary tract health. They are low in potassium and can be included in moderation in kidney-friendly juices. Cranberries add a zesty kick to your blends.

12. Beets:

Nutritional Content: Beets are a unique addition, offering natural sweetness and vibrant color to juices. They contain nitrates that may contribute to blood pressure regulation. Beets are moderate in potassium and can be part of kidney-friendly juicing.

CHAPTER 5

Juicing Techniques

Consider these juicing tips and techniques that elevate the art of creating delicious and nutrient-packed elixirs for kidney health.

1. Purchasing Fresh and Quality Produce:

The foundation of a great juice lies in the quality of your ingredients. Choose fresh, ripe fruits and vegetables to ensure optimal flavor and nutritional content. Consider organic options when possible to minimize exposure to pesticides.

2. Washing Thoroughly:

Before juicing, thoroughly wash all produce to remove dirt, pesticides, and contaminants. Even if you don't consume the peel, contaminants on the skin can transfer to the juice during the juicing process.

3. Balanced Variety:

Achieve a balance of flavors and nutrients by incorporating a variety of fruits and vegetables. This not only enhances the taste but also ensures a diverse array of vitamins, minerals, and antioxidants.

4. Experiment with Flavors:

They say the spice of life is experimentation. Mix sweet fruits with leafy greens, add a hint of citrus for brightness, or include a touch of ginger or herbs for a unique twist. Experimentation can lead to discovering your favorite concoctions.

5. Peel Wisely:

While some fruits and vegetables can be juiced with their peels, others may have bitter or tough peels that are better removed. For example, consider peeling citrus fruits and be mindful of the peel thickness on cucumbers.

6. Watch Your Portions:

Juicing can concentrate the sugars from fruits, so be mindful of portion sizes, especially if you're watching your sugar intake. Adding more vegetables than fruits helps keep the sugar content at moderate.

7. Incorporate Greens:

Leafy greens like kale and spinach are nutrient powerhouses and can be excellent additions to your juices. Start with milder greens if you're new to juicing greens and gradually increase the quantity.

8. Rotate Ingredients:

Vary your ingredients regularly to ensure a broad spectrum of nutrients. Rotating fruits and vegetables also helps prevent potential sensitivities or allergies that can arise from consuming the same foods daily.

9. Juice Immediately:

To preserve the freshness and nutritional content of your juice, consume it immediately after juicing. Exposure to air and light can lead to oxidation, which may reduce the potency of certain nutrients.

10. Clean Your Juicer Promptly:

Cleaning your juicer immediately after use prevents pulp and residue from drying, making the cleaning process easier. Most juicers come with dishwasher-safe parts for convenient cleaning.

Best Equipment for Juicing: Choosing Your Juicer

Selecting the right juicer is crucial for a seamless and enjoyable juicing experience. The type of juicer you choose depends on your preferences, the types of produce you plan to juice, and your budget. Here are three commonly used juicers:

1. Centrifugal Juicers:

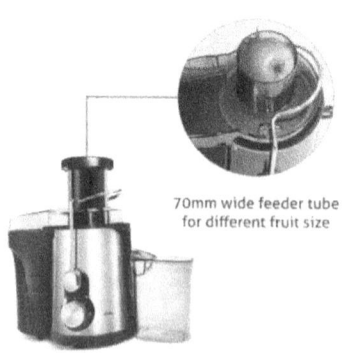

70mm wide feeder tube for different fruit size

Pros: Fast juicing process, suitable for hard fruits and vegetables, generally more affordable.

Cons: May produce heat that can affect nutrient content, less efficient with leafy greens.

2. Masticating Juicers (Cold Press or Slow Juicers):

Pros: Slow and gentle juicing process that retains more nutrients, efficient with leafy greens, can also make nut milks and sorbets.

Cons: Slower compared to centrifugal juicers, typically higher price point.

3. Twin Gear Juicers:

Pros: Efficient at extracting juice, retains high nutrient levels, versatile for various produce.

Cons: Higher cost, more complex assembly and cleaning process.

CHAPTER 6

Recipes for Kidney Health

Juice Recipe 1: Kidney Cleanser

Ingredients:

- ❖ 1 cucumber
- ❖ 1 cup watermelon cubes
- ❖ 1/2 cup blueberries
- ❖ 1 small beet, peeled
- ❖ Handful of fresh mint leaves

Instructions:

1. Wash all ingredients thoroughly.
2. Cut cucumber and beet into smaller pieces for easier juicing.
3. Juice all ingredients together.
4. Stir well and pour into a glass over ice.
5. Garnish with a sprig of mint for a refreshing touch.

Juice Recipe 2: Berry Bliss

Ingredients:

- ❖ 1 cup of mixed berries (blueberries, strawberries, Raspberries)
- ❖ 1 apple, cored
- ❖ 1/2 cup red grapes
- ❖ 1 handful spinach
- ❖ 1 teaspoon chia seeds (optional)

Instructions:

1. Wash all ingredients.
2. Remove stems from berries and core the apple.
3. Juice all ingredients, including the chia seeds if desired.
4. Mix well and enjoy the burst of berry flavors.

Juice Recipe 3: Citrus Delight

Ingredients:

- ❖ 2 oranges, peeled
- ❖ 1/2 lemon, peeled
- ❖ 1 carrot
- ❖ 1-inch piece of ginger

❖ 1 tablespoon fresh turmeric (or 1/2 teaspoon ground turmeric)

Instructions:

1. Peel oranges and lemon.
2. Cut carrot into smaller pieces.
3. Juice all ingredients together, including ginger and turmeric.
4. Stir well and savor the zesty citrus infusion.
5. Highlighting Specific Recipes for Different Kidney Conditions

For those with Chronic Kidney Disease (CKD):

Juice Recipe 4: Green Kidney Booster

Ingredients:

❖ 1 cup kale
❖ 1/2 cucumber
❖ 1 green apple, cored
❖ 1 celery stalk
❖ 1/2 lemon, peeled

Instructions:

1. Wash and prepare all ingredients.
2. Juice the kale, cucumber, apple, celery, and lemon together.
3. Mix well and pour into a glass.
4. A nutrient-dense, kidney-friendly green elixir is ready to enjoy.

For those with Hypertension:

Juice Recipe 5: Beet and Berry Blood Pressure Balancer

Ingredients:

- ❖ 1 small beet, peeled
- ❖ 1 cup mixed berries (blueberries, strawberries)
- ❖ 1/2 cucumber
- ❖ 1 tablespoon flaxseeds (optional)

Instructions:

1. Wash and peel the beet.
2. Prepare the berries and cucumber.
3. Juice all ingredients, including flaxseeds if desired.

4. Stir well and savor this blood pressure-balancing blend.

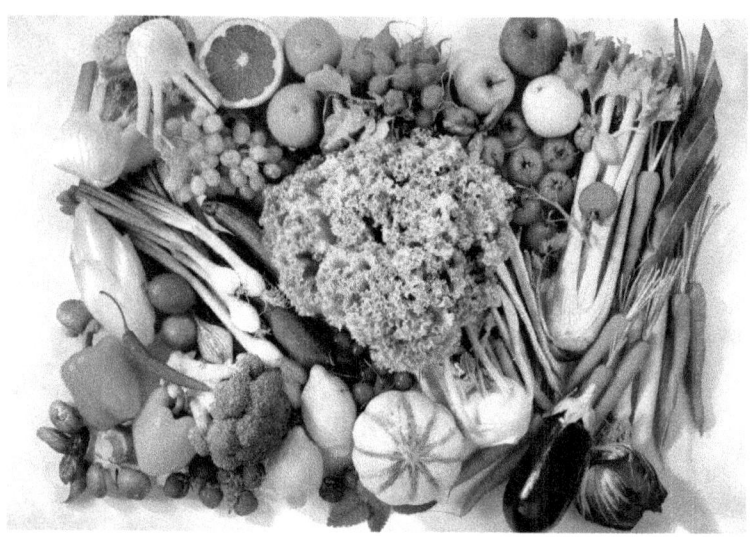

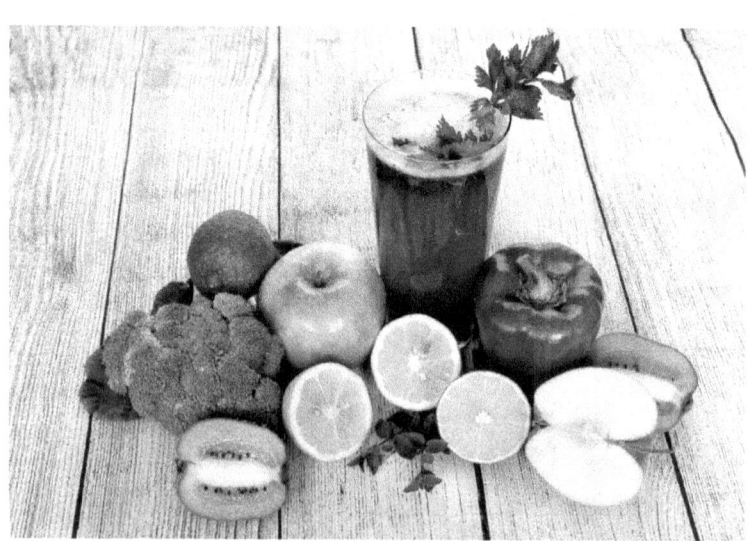

CHAPTER 7

Incorporating Herbs and Supplements

Herbs and Supplements for Kidney Health:

Dandelion Root:

Known for its diuretic properties, dandelion root may help promote kidney function. It can be brewed into tea or added as a supplement.

Nettle Leaf:

Nettle leaf is rich in antioxidants and may have anti-inflammatory effects. This can be taken as a supplement or as tea.

Turmeric:

The active compound in turmeric has anti-inflammatory properties. Use fresh turmeric in juices or consider turmeric supplements.

Ginger:

Ginger has anti-inflammatory and antioxidant properties. Fresh ginger can be added to juices or consumed as a supplement.

Guidance on Safe and Effective Usage of the above mentioned herbs and supplements:

Before incorporating herbs or supplements, consult with a healthcare professional, especially if you have pre-existing health conditions or are on medications. Do this in little portions and monitor your intakes for any adverse reactions, be aware of potential interactions between herbs/supplements and medications.

CHAPTER 8

Lifestyle Tips for Kidney Health

Regular Exercise:

Engage in moderate exercise, such as walking or swimming, to support overall kidney function and cardiovascular health.

Stress Management:

Practice stress-reducing activities like meditation, deep breathing, or yoga to promote emotional well-being, as chronic stress can impact kidney health.

Adequate Sleep:

Ensure you have 7-9 hours of quality sleep per night to support overall health, including kidney function and repair.

CHAPTER 9

Consulting with Healthcare Professionals

Healthcare professionals serve as advocates for kidney health, guiding individuals on a path that combines medical expertise with personal empowerment. As individuals navigate the realm of dietary choices, juicing, and lifestyle adjustments, the collaborative relationship with healthcare providers becomes a beacon of support and knowledge.

Consultation with a healthcare professional is non-negotiable. Nephrologists, dietitians, and other healthcare providers bring specialized knowledge that is indispensable in crafting a tailored approach.

Individualized Assessment:

Healthcare professionals conduct a comprehensive assessment of an individual's health history, current medical conditions, medications, and lab results. This holistic understanding forms the foundation for personalized recommendations.

Understanding Dietary Restrictions:

For individuals with kidney conditions, dietary restrictions may be necessary to manage factors such as protein, phosphorus, potassium, and sodium intake. Healthcare professionals can guide individuals in navigating these restrictions while ensuring adequate nutrition.

Medication Interactions:

Some herbs and supplements used in juicing may interact with medications. Healthcare professionals possess the expertise to identify potential interactions and make adjustments to medication regimens as needed.

Monitoring Health Parameters:

Regular monitoring of kidney function through blood tests is essential. Healthcare professionals track changes, assess the impact of dietary modifications, and make adjustments accordingly.

Addressing Underlying Conditions:

Conditions like diabetes and hypertension, common contributors to kidney issues, often require specific dietary management. Healthcare professionals can provide targeted

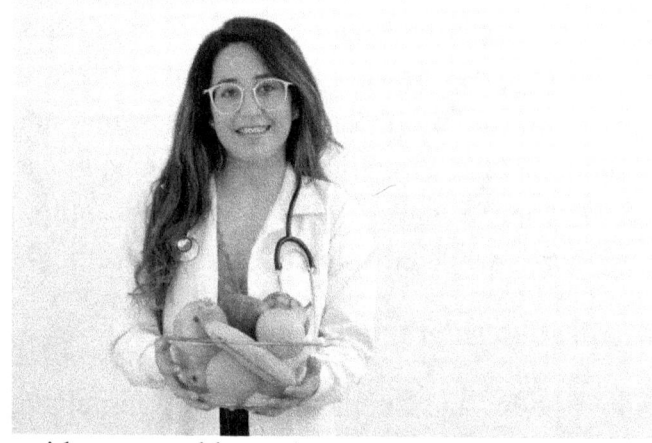

guidance to address these underlying concerns.

CHAPTER FINALE

Success Stories

Hurray!!! You made it to the final chapter of this amazing piece, this chapter remain my favorite chapter; the success stories of me and people who read this book to the very end. I hope you derive some form of encouragement and resilience from the stories of others. For the purpose of privacy, random names would be used as a representation of persons involved.

Success Story 1: Rediscovering Vitality with Juicing

Sarah, a vibrant individual who faced the challenges of Chronic Kidney Disease (CKD) with resilience and determination. Battling fatigue, Sarah embarked on a journey to rejuvenate her kidney health through juicing. By incorporating a variety of kidney-friendly fruits and vegetables, such as cucumbers, berries, and leafy greens, Sarah experienced a transformative surge in energy.

Her daily ritual included a hydrating cucumber and watermelon blend infused with mint, providing essential nutrients while maintaining hydration. Sarah also crafted antioxidant-rich juices with berries, contributing to the management of oxidative stress—a key concern for those with CKD.

Regular check-ups with her healthcare team reflected improvements in her kidney function. With the support of her nephrologist and a personalized juicing plan, Sarah not only slowed the progression of CKD but also regained a sense of vitality that she thought was lost. Her success story illustrates the empowering synergy of juicing and healthcare in fostering kidney resilience.

Success Story 2: Managing Hypertension through Flavorful Juices

John, a middle-aged professional, found himself grappling with hypertension, a condition known to strain the kidneys. Determined to take control of his health, John embraced a lifestyle overhaul that prominently featured juicing. His concoctions included a dynamic mix of beets, berries, and leafy greens, carefully crafted to support blood pressure regulation and kidney health.

The integration of juicing into his daily routine not only became a delightful sensory experience but also a therapeutic endeavor. John's journey, guided by collaborative efforts with his healthcare team, showcased a significant reduction in blood pressure readings over time.

Regular communication with his healthcare provider allowed for adjustments to his juicing plan as needed. John's success story underscores the symbiotic relationship between mindful juicing and medical guidance in managing conditions that impact kidney health.

Success Story 3: Kidney Rejuvenation through Nutrient-Packed Elixirs

James, a fitness enthusiast, discovered the potential of juicing in supporting kidney health during his battle with acute kidney injury. Recognizing the need for a nutrient-dense approach, James incorporated a kaleidoscope of ingredients into his juices, including kale, spinach, citrus, and ginger.

These carefully curated elixirs not only provided a burst of flavor but also delivered a concentrated dose of vitamins and minerals. James's commitment to his juicing routine, complemented by regular consultations with his healthcare team, contributed to a remarkable recovery.

James's journey emphasizes the resilience of the kidneys when provided with the right nourishment. His success showcases the healing potential of nutrient-packed juices in the context of acute kidney challenges.

Conclusion

A Symphony of Wellness through Juicing

In the tapestry of kidney health, these success stories illuminate the transformative power of juicing when harmonized with professional healthcare guidance. From managing chronic conditions to supporting recovery from acute challenges, juicing emerges as a vibrant thread that weaves through the stories of Sarah, John, and James.

Key Pointers:

Personalized Approaches Matter:

Each individual's journey is unique. Tailoring juicing plans to align with specific health conditions and preferences is key to success.

Collaboration with Healthcare Professionals:

Success stories underscore the importance of collaborative efforts with healthcare teams. Regular check-ups, open communication, and adjustments based on professional guidance enhance the effectiveness of juicing for kidney health.

Nutrient Density and Variety:

Nutrient-packed juices, enriched with a variety of fruits, vegetables, and herbs, provide a holistic approach to kidney health. The diverse nutritional profiles contribute to overall well-being.

Holistic Wellness:

Beyond juicing, success stories emphasize the integration of lifestyle changes, stress management, and adequate sleep. A holistic approach nurtures not only kidney health but also the overall vitality of individuals.

Take Proactive Steps:

As we conclude these narratives of triumph, let them serve as an invitation to take proactive steps toward maintaining kidney health. Whether you're navigating chronic conditions, hypertension, or aiming for general well-being, the synergy of juicing and healthcare expertise offers a path to resilience.

Consult with healthcare professionals for personalized guidance, and embark on a journey where the symphony of wellness plays a beautiful tune. Through mindful choices and collaborative care, you have the power to script your own success story—one where kidney health thrives, and vitality blossoms.

Thank You!!!